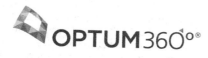

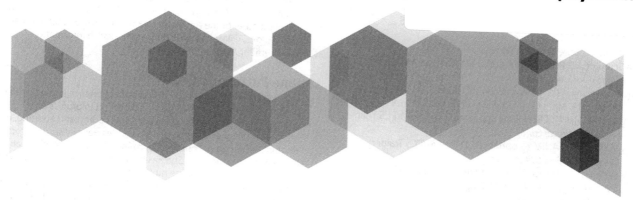

# 2018

# ICD-10-CM Professional for Physicians

The complete official code set
Codes valid October 1, 2017 through September 30, 2018

**POWER UP YOUR CODING** with Optum360, your trusted
coding partner for 32 years. **Visit optum360coding.com.**

## Publisher's Notice

The *ICD-10-CM Professional for Physicians: The Complete Official Code Set* is designed to be an accurate and authoritative source regarding coding and every reasonable effort has been made to ensure accuracy and completeness of the content. However, Optum360 makes no guarantee, warranty, or representation that this publication is accurate, complete or without errors. It is understood that Optum360 is not rendering any legal or other professional services or advice in this publication and that Optum360 bears no liability for any results or consequences that may arise from the use of this book.

## Acknowledgments

Lauri Gray, RHIT, CPC, AHIMA-approved ICD-10-CM/PCS Trainer, *Product Manager*

Karen Schmidt, BSN, *Technical Director*

Anita Schmidt, BS, RHIT, AHIMA-approved ICD-10-CM/PCS Trainer, *Clinical Technical Editor*

Leanne Patterson, CPC, *Clinical Technical Editor*

Anne Kenney, BA, MBA, CCA, CCS, *Clinical Technical Editor*

Karen Krawzik, RHIT, CCS, AHIMA-approved ICD-10-CM/PCS Trainer, *Clinical Technical Editor*

Peggy Willard, CCS, AHIMA-approved ICD-10-CM/PCS Trainer, *Clinical Technical Editor*

Dr. Vikas Kumar, BHMS, CPC, CPC-H, *Clinical Technical Editor*

Stacy Perry, *Manager, Desktop Publishing*

Lisa Singley, *Project Manager*

Tracy Betzler, *Senior Desktop Publishing Specialist*

Hope M. Dunn, *Senior Desktop Publishing Specialist*

Katie Russell, *Desktop Publishing Specialist*

Kate Holden, *Editor*

## Our Commitment to Accuracy

Optum360 is committed to producing accurate and reliable materials.

To report corrections, please visit www.optum360coding.com/accuracy or email accuracy@optum.com. You can also reach customer service by calling 1.800.464.3649, option 1.

## Anita Schmidt, BS, RHIT, AHIMA-approved ICD-10-CM/PCS Trainer

Ms. Schmidt has expertise in Level I Adult and Pediatric Trauma hospital coding, specializing in ICD-9-CM, ICD-10-CM/PCS, DRG, and CPT coding. Her experience includes analysis of medical record documentation, assignment of ICD-10-CM and PCS codes, DRG validation, as well as CPT code assignments for same-day surgery cases. She has conducted coding training and auditing, including DRG validation, conducted electronic health record training, and worked with clinical documentation specialists to identify documentation needs and potential areas for physician education. Most recently she has been developing content for resource and educational products related to ICD-10-CM and ICD-10-PCS. Ms. Schmidt is an AHIMA-approved ICD-10-CM/PCS trainer, and is an active member of the American Health Information Management Association (AHIMA) and the Minnesota Health Information Management Association (MHIMA).

## Leanne Patterson, CPC

Ms. Patterson has more than 10 years of experience in the health care profession. She has an extensive background in professional component coding, with expertise in E/M coding and auditing, and HIPAA compliance. Her experience includes general surgery coding, serving as director of compliance, conducting chart-to-claim audits and physician education. She has been responsible for coding and denial management in large multispecialty physician practices, and most recently served as a practice manager where she supervised implementation of a new EHR system. Ms. Patterson is credentialed by the American Academy of Professional Coders (AAPC) as a Certified Professional Coder (CPC).

# Contents

# Contents

## ICD-10-CM Official Preface

This FY 2018 update of the International Statistical Classification of Diseases and Related Health Problems, 10th revision, Clinical Modification (ICD-10-CM) is being published by the United States government in recognition of its responsibility to promulgate this classification throughout the United States for morbidity coding. The International Statistical Classification of Diseases and Related Health Problems, 10th Revision (ICD-10), published by the World Health Organization (WHO), is the foundation of ICD-10-CM. ICD-10 continues to be the classification used in cause-of-death coding in the United States. The ICD-10-CM is comparable with the ICD-10. The WHO Collaborating Center for the Family of International Classifications in North America, housed at the Centers for Disease Control and Prevention's National Center for Health Statistics (NCHS), has responsibility for the implementation of ICD and other WHO-FIC classifications and serves as a liaison with the WHO, fulfilling international obligations for comparable classifications and the national health data needs of the United States. The historical background of ICD and ICD-10 can be found in the Introduction to the International Classification of Diseases and Related Health Problems (ICD-10), 2010, World Health Organization, Geneva, Switzerland.

ICD-10-CM is the United States' clinical modification of the World Health Organization's ICD-10. The term "clinical" is used to emphasize the modification's intent: to serve as a useful tool in the area of classification of morbidity data for indexing of health records, medical care review, and ambulatory and other health care programs, as well as for basic health statistics. To describe the clinical picture of the patient the codes must be more precise than those needed only for statistical groupings and trend analysis.

## Characteristics of ICD-10-CM

ICD-10-CM far exceeds its predecessors in the number of concepts and codes provided. The disease classification has been expanded to include health-related conditions and to provide greater specificity at the sixth and seventh character level. The sixth and seventh characters are not optional and are intended for use in recording the information documented in the clinical record.

ICD-10-CM extensions, interpretations, modifications, addenda, or errata other than those approved by the Centers for Disease Control and Prevention are not to be considered official and should not be utilized. Continuous maintenance of the ICD-10- CM is the responsibility of the aforementioned agencies. However, because the ICD-10- CM represents the best in contemporary thinking of clinicians, nosologists, epidemiologists, and statisticians from both public and private sectors, when future modifications are considered, advice will be sought from all stakeholders.

All official authorized addenda since the last complete update (October 1, 2017) have been included in this revision. For more detailed information please see the complete official authorized addenda to ICD-10-CM, including the "ICD-10-CM Official Guidelines for Coding and Reporting," and a description of the ICD-10-CM updating and maintenance process.

# What's New for 2018

## Official Updates

The National Center for Health Statistics (NCHS), a section of the Centers for Disease Control and Prevention (CDC), is the agency charged with maintaining and updating ICD-10-CM. The 2018 official addendum was posted to the Centers for Medicare and Medicaid Services (CMS) website on June 13, 2017, identifying the changes to the ICD-10-CM code set for fiscal 2018. A summary of changes is provided below:

- 360 new codes added

- 226 code descriptions revised

- 34 codes changed from valid to invalid

**Note:** Validity changes are the result of new codes being added to the classification, changing a previously valid code to an invalid code, creating a new subcategory.

| | |
|---|---|
| A04.7 | Enterocolitis due to Clostridium difficile |
| C96.2 | Malignant mast cell tumor |
| D47.0 | Histiocytic and mast cell tumors of uncertain behavior |
| E85.8 | Other amyloidosis |
| H54.0 | Blindness, both eyes |
| H54.11 | Blindness, right eye, low vision left eye |
| H54.12 | Blindness, left eye, low vision right eye |
| H54.2 | Low vision, both eyes |
| H54.41 | Blindness, right eye, normal vision left eye |
| H54.42 | Blindness, left eye, normal vision right eye |
| H54.51 | Low vision, right eye, normal vision left eye |
| H54.52 | Low vision, left eye, normal vision right eye |
| I27.2 | Other secondary pulmonary hypertension |
| K06.0 | Gingival recession |
| K56.5 | Intestinal adhesions [bands] with obstruction (postprocedural) (postinfection) |
| K56.60 | Unspecified intestinal obstruction |
| K56.69 | Other intestinal obstruction |
| K91.3 | Postprocedural intestinal obstruction |
| M48.06 | Spinal stenosis, lumbar region |
| N63 | Unspecified lump in breast |
| O00.10 | Tubal pregnancy without intrauterine pregnancy |
| O00.11 | Tubal pregnancy with intrauterine pregnancy |
| O00.20 | Ovarian pregnancy without intrauterine pregnancy |
| O00.21 | Ovarian pregnancy with intrauterine pregnancy |
| P29.3 | Persistent fetal circulation |
| P83.8 | Other specified conditions of integument specific to newborn |
| P91.8 | Other specified disturbances of cerebral status of newborn |
| Q53.11 | Abdominal testis, unilateral |
| Q53.21 | Abdominal testis, bilateral |
| T07 | Unspecified multiple injuries |
| T14.8 | Other injury of unspecified body region |
| T14.90 | Injury, unspecified |
| T14.91 | Suicide attempt |
| Z36 | Encounter for antenatal screening of mother [end indent] |

- 122 codes deleted from the classification

| | |
|---|---|
| S06.1X7D | Traumatic cerebral edema with loss of consciousness of any duration with death due to brain injury prior to regaining consciousness, subsequent encounter |
| S06.1X7S | Traumatic cerebral edema with loss of consciousness of any duration with death due to brain injury prior to regaining consciousness, sequela |
| S06.1X8D | Traumatic cerebral edema with loss of consciousness of any duration with death due to other cause prior to regaining consciousness, subsequent encounter |
| S06.1X8S | Traumatic cerebral edema with loss of consciousness of any duration with death due to other cause prior to regaining consciousness, sequela |
| S06.2X7D | Diffuse traumatic brain injury with loss of consciousness of any duration with death due to brain injury prior to regaining consciousness, subsequent encounter |
| S06.2X7S | Diffuse traumatic brain injury with loss of consciousness of any duration with death due to brain injury prior to regaining consciousness, sequela |
| S06.2X8D | Diffuse traumatic brain injury with loss of consciousness of any duration with death due to other cause prior to regaining consciousness, subsequent encounter |
| S06.2X8S | Diffuse traumatic brain injury with loss of consciousness of any duration with death due to other cause prior to regaining consciousness, sequela |
| S06.307D | Unspecified focal traumatic brain injury with loss of consciousness of any duration with death due to brain injury prior to regaining consciousness, subsequent encounter |
| S06.307S | Unspecified focal traumatic brain injury with loss of consciousness of any duration with death due to brain injury prior to regaining consciousness, sequela |
| S06.308D | Unspecified focal traumatic brain injury with loss of consciousness of any duration with death due to other cause prior to regaining consciousness, subsequent encounter |
| S06.308S | Unspecified focal traumatic brain injury with loss of consciousness of any duration with death due to other cause prior to regaining consciousness, sequela |
| S06.317D | Contusion and laceration of right cerebrum with loss of consciousness of any duration with death due to brain injury prior to regaining consciousness, subsequent encounter |
| S06.317S | Contusion and laceration of right cerebrum with loss of consciousness of any duration with death due to brain injury prior to regaining consciousness, sequela |
| S06.318D | Contusion and laceration of right cerebrum with loss of consciousness of any duration with death due to other cause prior to regaining consciousness, subsequent encounter |
| S06.318S | Contusion and laceration of right cerebrum with loss of consciousness of any duration with death due to other cause prior to regaining consciousness, sequela |
| S06.327D | Contusion and laceration of left cerebrum with loss of consciousness of any duration with death due to brain injury prior to regaining consciousness, subsequent encounter |
| S06.327S | Contusion and laceration of left cerebrum with loss of consciousness of any duration with death due to brain injury prior to regaining consciousness, sequela |
| S06.328D | Contusion and laceration of left cerebrum with loss of consciousness of any duration with death due to other cause prior to regaining consciousness, subsequent encounter |
| S06.328S | Contusion and laceration of left cerebrum with loss of consciousness of any duration with death due to other cause prior to regaining consciousness, sequela |
| S06.337D | Contusion and laceration of cerebrum, unspecified, with loss of consciousness of any duration with death due to brain injury prior to regaining consciousness, subsequent encounter |
| S06.337S | Contusion and laceration of cerebrum, unspecified, with loss of consciousness of any duration with death due to brain injury prior to regaining consciousness, sequela |
| S06.338D | Contusion and laceration of cerebrum, unspecified, with loss of consciousness of any duration with death due to other cause prior to regaining consciousness, subsequent encounter |
| S06.338S | Contusion and laceration of cerebrum, unspecified, with loss of consciousness of any duration with death due to other cause prior to regaining consciousness, sequela |
| S06.347D | Traumatic hemorrhage of right cerebrum with loss of consciousness of any duration with death due to brain injury prior to regaining consciousness, subsequent encounter |

S06.347S  Traumatic hemorrhage of right cerebrum with loss of consciousness of any duration with death due to brain injury prior to regaining consciousness, sequela

S06.348D  Traumatic hemorrhage of right cerebrum with loss of consciousness of any duration with death due to other cause prior to regaining consciousness, subsequent encounter

S06.348S  Traumatic hemorrhage of right cerebrum with loss of consciousness of any duration with death due to other cause prior to regaining consciousness, sequela

S06.357D  Traumatic hemorrhage of left cerebrum with loss of consciousness of any duration with death due to brain injury prior to regaining consciousness, subsequent encounter

S06.357S  Traumatic hemorrhage of left cerebrum with loss of consciousness of any duration with death due to brain injury prior to regaining consciousness, sequela

S06.358D  Traumatic hemorrhage of left cerebrum with loss of consciousness of any duration with death due to other cause prior to regaining consciousness, subsequent encounter

S06.358S  Traumatic hemorrhage of left cerebrum with loss of consciousness of any duration with death due to other cause prior to regaining consciousness, sequela

S06.367D  Traumatic hemorrhage of cerebrum, unspecified, with loss of consciousness of any duration with death due to brain injury prior to regaining consciousness, subsequent encounter

S06.367S  Traumatic hemorrhage of cerebrum, unspecified, with loss of consciousness of any duration with death due to brain injury prior to regaining consciousness, sequela

S06.368D  Traumatic hemorrhage of cerebrum, unspecified, with loss of consciousness of any duration with death due to other cause prior to regaining consciousness, subsequent encounter

S06.368S  Traumatic hemorrhage of cerebrum, unspecified, with loss of consciousness of any duration with death due to other cause prior to regaining consciousness, sequela

S06.377D  Contusion, laceration, and hemorrhage of cerebellum with loss of consciousness of any duration with death due to brain injury prior to regaining consciousness, subsequent encounter

S06.377S  Contusion, laceration, and hemorrhage of cerebellum with loss of consciousness of any duration with death due to brain injury prior to regaining consciousness, sequela

S06.378D  Contusion, laceration, and hemorrhage of cerebellum with loss of consciousness of any duration with death due to other cause prior to regaining consciousness, subsequent encounter

S06.378S  Contusion, laceration, and hemorrhage of cerebellum with loss of consciousness of any duration with death due to other cause prior to regaining consciousness, sequela

S06.387D  Contusion, laceration, and hemorrhage of brainstem with loss of consciousness of any duration with death due to brain injury prior to regaining consciousness, subsequent encounter

S06.387S  Contusion, laceration, and hemorrhage of brainstem with loss of consciousness of any duration with death due to brain injury prior to regaining consciousness, sequela

S06.388D  Contusion, laceration, and hemorrhage of brainstem with loss of consciousness of any duration with death due to other cause prior to regaining consciousness, subsequent encounter

S06.388S  Contusion, laceration, and hemorrhage of brainstem with loss of consciousness of any duration with death due to other cause prior to regaining consciousness, sequela

S06.4X7D  Epidural hemorrhage with loss of consciousness of any duration with death due to brain injury prior to regaining consciousness, subsequent encounter

S06.4X7S  Epidural hemorrhage with loss of consciousness of any duration with death due to brain injury prior to regaining consciousness, sequela

S06.4X8D  Epidural hemorrhage with loss of consciousness of any duration with death due to other causes prior to regaining consciousness, subsequent encounter

S06.4X8S  Epidural hemorrhage with loss of consciousness of any duration with death due to other causes prior to regaining consciousness, sequela

S06.5X7D  Traumatic subdural hemorrhage with loss of consciousness of any duration with death due to brain injury before regaining consciousness, subsequent encounter

S06.5X7S  Traumatic subdural hemorrhage with loss of consciousness of any duration with death due to brain injury before regaining consciousness, sequela

S06.5X8D  Traumatic subdural hemorrhage with loss of consciousness of any duration with death due to other cause before regaining consciousness, subsequent encounter

S06.5X8S  Traumatic subdural hemorrhage with loss of consciousness of any duration with death due to other cause before regaining consciousness, sequela

S06.6X7D  Traumatic subarachnoid hemorrhage with loss of consciousness of any duration with death due to brain injury prior to regaining consciousness, subsequent encounter

S06.6X7S  Traumatic subarachnoid hemorrhage with loss of consciousness of any duration with death due to brain injury prior to regaining consciousness, sequela

S06.6X8D  Traumatic subarachnoid hemorrhage with loss of consciousness of any duration with death due to other cause prior to regaining consciousness, subsequent encounter

S06.6X8S  Traumatic subarachnoid hemorrhage with loss of consciousness of any duration with death due to other cause prior to regaining consciousness, sequela

S06.817D  Injury of right internal carotid artery, intracranial portion, not elsewhere classified with loss of consciousness of any duration with death due to brain injury prior to regaining consciousness, subsequent encounter

S06.817S  Injury of right internal carotid artery, intracranial portion, not elsewhere classified with loss of consciousness of any duration with death due to brain injury prior to regaining consciousness, sequela

S06.818D  Injury of right internal carotid artery, intracranial portion, not elsewhere classified with loss of consciousness of any duration with death due to other cause prior to regaining consciousness, subsequent encounter

S06.818S  Injury of right internal carotid artery, intracranial portion, not elsewhere classified with loss of consciousness of any duration with death due to other cause prior to regaining consciousness, sequela

S06.827D  Injury of left internal carotid artery, intracranial portion, not elsewhere classified with loss of consciousness of any duration with death due to brain injury prior to regaining consciousness, subsequent encounter

S06.827S  Injury of left internal carotid artery, intracranial portion, not elsewhere classified with loss of consciousness of any duration with death due to brain injury prior to regaining consciousness, sequela

S06.828D  Injury of left internal carotid artery, intracranial portion, not elsewhere classified with loss of consciousness of any duration with death due to other cause prior to regaining consciousness, subsequent encounter

S06.828S  Injury of left internal carotid artery, intracranial portion, not elsewhere classified with loss of consciousness of any duration with death due to other cause prior to regaining consciousness, sequela

S06.897D  Other specified intracranial injury with loss of consciousness of any duration with death due to brain injury prior to regaining consciousness, subsequent encounter

S06.897S  Other specified intracranial injury with loss of consciousness of any duration with death due to brain injury prior to regaining consciousness, sequela

S06.898D  Other specified intracranial injury with loss of consciousness of any duration with death due to other cause prior to regaining consciousness, subsequent encounter

S06.898S  Other specified intracranial injury with loss of consciousness of any duration with death due to other cause prior to regaining consciousness, sequela

S06.9X7D  Unspecified intracranial injury with loss of consciousness of any duration with death due to brain injury prior to regaining consciousness, subsequent encounter

S06.9X7S  Unspecified intracranial injury with loss of consciousness of any duration with death due to brain injury prior to regaining consciousness, sequela

S06.9X8D  Unspecified intracranial injury with loss of consciousness of any duration with death due to other cause prior to regaining consciousness, subsequent encounter

S06.9X8S  Unspecified intracranial injury with loss of consciousness of any duration with death due to other cause prior to regaining consciousness, sequela

S63.13  Subluxation and dislocation of proximal interphalangeal joint of thumb

S63.131  Subluxation of proximal interphalangeal joint of right thumb

S63.131A  Subluxation of proximal interphalangeal joint of right thumb, initial encounter

S63.131D  Subluxation of proximal interphalangeal joint of right thumb, subsequent encounter

S63.131S  Subluxation of proximal interphalangeal joint of right thumb, sequela

S63.132  Subluxation of proximal interphalangeal joint of left thumb

S63.132A  Subluxation of proximal interphalangeal joint of left thumb, initial encounter

S63.132D  Subluxation of proximal interphalangeal joint of left thumb, subsequent encounter

S63.132S  Subluxation of proximal interphalangeal joint of left thumb, sequela

S63.133  Subluxation of proximal interphalangeal joint of unspecified thumb

S63.133A  Subluxation of proximal interphalangeal joint of unspecified thumb, initial encounter

S63.133D  Subluxation of proximal interphalangeal joint of unspecified thumb, subsequent encounter

S63.133S  Subluxation of proximal interphalangeal joint of unspecified thumb, sequela

S63.134  Dislocation of proximal interphalangeal joint of right thumb

S63.134A  Dislocation of proximal interphalangeal joint of right thumb, initial encounter

S63.134D  Dislocation of proximal interphalangeal joint of right thumb, subsequent encounter

S63.134S  Dislocation of proximal interphalangeal joint of right thumb, sequela

S63.135  Dislocation of proximal interphalangeal joint of left thumb

S63.135A  Dislocation of proximal interphalangeal joint of left thumb, initial encounter

S63.135D  Dislocation of proximal interphalangeal joint of left thumb, subsequent encounter

S63.135S  Dislocation of proximal interphalangeal joint of left thumb, sequela

S63.136  Dislocation of proximal interphalangeal joint of unspecified thumb

S63.136A  Dislocation of proximal interphalangeal joint of unspecified thumb, initial encounter

S63.136D  Dislocation of proximal interphalangeal joint of unspecified thumb, subsequent encounter

S63.136S  Dislocation of proximal interphalangeal joint of unspecified thumb, sequela

S63.14  Subluxation and dislocation of distal interphalangeal joint of thumb

S63.141  Subluxation of distal interphalangeal joint of right thumb

S63.141A  Subluxation of distal interphalangeal joint of right thumb, initial encounter

S63.141D  Subluxation of distal interphalangeal joint of right thumb, subsequent encounter

S63.141S  Subluxation of distal interphalangeal joint of right thumb, sequela

S63.142  Subluxation of distal interphalangeal joint of left thumb

S63.142A  Subluxation of distal interphalangeal joint of left thumb, initial encounter

S63.142D  Subluxation of distal interphalangeal joint of left thumb, subsequent encounter

S63.142S  Subluxation of distal interphalangeal joint of left thumb, sequela

S63.143  Subluxation of distal interphalangeal joint of unspecified thumb

S63.143A  Subluxation of distal interphalangeal joint of unspecified thumb, initial encounter

S63.143D  Subluxation of distal interphalangeal joint of unspecified thumb, subsequent encounter

S63.143S  Subluxation of distal interphalangeal joint of unspecified thumb, sequela

S63.144  Dislocation of distal interphalangeal joint of right thumb

S63.144A  Dislocation of distal interphalangeal joint of right thumb, initial encounter

S63.144D  Dislocation of distal interphalangeal joint of right thumb, subsequent encounter

S63.144S  Dislocation of distal interphalangeal joint of right thumb, sequela

S63.145  Dislocation of distal interphalangeal joint of left thumb

S63.145A  Dislocation of distal interphalangeal joint of left thumb, initial encounter

S63.145D  Dislocation of distal interphalangeal joint of left thumb, subsequent encounter

S63.145S  Dislocation of distal interphalangeal joint of left thumb, sequela

S63.146  Dislocation of distal interphalangeal joint of unspecified thumb

S63.146A  Dislocation of distal interphalangeal joint of unspecified thumb, initial encounter

S63.146D  Dislocation of distal interphalangeal joint of unspecified thumb, subsequent encounter

S63.146S  Dislocation of distal interphalangeal joint of unspecified thumb, sequela

## Proprietary Updates

The following proprietary features have also been added:

- 150+ new definitions that describe, in lay terms, a specific condition or disease process

- 50+ new illustrations

- Updated *AHA Coding Clinic* references through second quarter 2017

- Updated pharmacology list

- New HCC icon identifying CMS hierarchical condition category (CMS-HCC) codes

- Updated coding examples in the chapter-specific guideline sections that are specific to the physician setting

# Introduction

## History of ICD-10-CM

The ICD-10-CM classification system was developed by the National Center for Health Statistics (NCHS) as a clinical modification to the ICD-10 system developed by the World Health Organization (WHO), primarily as a unique system for use in the United States for morbidity and mortality reporting. Although ICD-10 replaced ICD-9 for use in coding and classifying mortality data from death certificates beginning January 1, 1999, ICD-10-CM implementation was postponed many years until legislation to replace ICD-9-CM, volumes 1 and 2, with ICD-10-CM was approved.

ICD-10 is the copyrighted product of the World Health Organization (WHO), which has authorized the development of a clinical modification (CM) of ICD-10 for use in the United States. However, all modifications to the ICD-10 must conform to WHO conventions for ICD. The development of ICD-10-CM included comprehensive evaluation by a Technical Advisory Panel and extensive consultation with physician groups, clinical coders, and other industry experts.

The ICD-10-CM draft and crosswalk between ICD-9-CM and ICD-10-CM were made available on the Centers for Medicare and Medicaid Services (CMS) website for public comment. The initial public comment period extended from December 1997 through February 1998. A field test for ICD-10-CM was conducted in the summer of 2003 jointly by the American Hospital Association (AHA) and the American Health Information Management Association (AHIMA). Public comments and suggestions were reviewed and additional modifications to ICD-10-CM were made. Revisions were made to ICD-10-CM based on the established update process for ICD-10-CM (the ICD-10-CM Coordination and Maintenance Committee) and the World Health Organization's ICD-10 (the Update and Revision Committee).

These revisions to ICD-10-CM have included:

- Information relevant to ambulatory and managed care encounters
- Expanded injury codes
- Creation of combination diagnosis/symptom codes to reduce the number of codes needed to fully describe a condition
- The addition of 6th and 7th character classifications
- Incorporation of common 4th and 5th character classifications
- Classifications specific to laterality
- Classification refinement for increased data granularity

This new structure allows for further expansion than was possible with the ICD-9-CM classification system.

The Department of Health and Human Services (HHS) published the final rule regarding the adoption of both ICD-10-CM and ICD-10-PCS in the January 16, 2009, *Federal Register* (45 CFR part 162 [CMS—0013—F]). The initial compliance date for implementation of ICD-10-CM and ICD-10-PCS as a replacement for ICD-9-CM was set at October 1, 2013. On April 17, 2012, the Department of Health and Human Services (HHS) released a notice to postpone the date by which certain health care entities have to comply with International Classification of Diseases, 10th Revision diagnosis and procedure codes (ICD-10). The compliance date for implementation of ICD-10-CM and ICD-10-PCS as a replacement for ICD-9-CM was changed to October 1, 2014. On April 1, 2014, Congress enacted the Protecting Access to Medicare Act of 2014, which contained a provision to delay the implementation of ICD-10-CM/PCS by at least one year, prohibiting the Department of Health and Human Services (HHS) from adopting the ICD-10-CM/PCS code sets as the mandatory standard until October 1, 2015. Eventually, the ICD-10-CM/PCS code sets were implemented in their entirety on October 1, 2015, and volumes 1 and 2 of ICD-9-CM were retired.

## ICD-10-CM: The Complete Official Code Set

*ICD-10-CM for Physicians: The Complete Official Code Set* 2018 edition includes many of the enhancements described below in direct response to requests from our subscribers. Users will find many of the conventions, icons, color bars, and other enhancements familiar since many of these features are similar to the hallmark color coding and symbols of our ICD-9-CM code books.

As you review the content, you will find the following:

- Optum360 Exclusive feature — Check Placeholder Alert symbol, indicating the need for one or more "filler" X character assignments in the 5th and/or 6th character position, in order to appropriately assign a required character in the 7th character position
- Optum360 Exclusive feature — Key word differentiation by the use of a green font that highlights the differentiating terms in similar code descriptions in a given category
- Optum360 Exclusive color coding, symbols, and footnotes that alert coders to coding and reimbursement issues, including the majority of the Medicare code edits
- Optum360 Exclusive feature — Exclusive *following* references and Check Additional Character symbol in the indexes. The *following* references (designed and used exclusively by Optum360) help coders locate those alphanumeric codes that are out of sequence in the tabular section.
- Optum360 Exclusive feature — Exclusive shaded guides in the index that help users easily follow the indent levels for the subterms under a main term
- Illustrations throughout the tabular list and at the back of the book that feature anatomy and terminology included in the ICD-10-CM classification system
- Optum360 Exclusive feature — Detailed Muscle/Tendon tables that correspond to codes in chapters 13 and 19
- The complete ICD-10-CM Official Guidelines for Coding and Reporting, published by the U.S. Department of Health and Human Services and approved by the cooperating parties (American Health Information Management Association, National Center for Health Statistics, Centers for Medicare and Medicaid Services, American Hospital Association)
- Optum360 Exclusive feature — Official chapter-specific guidelines with coding examples at the beginning of each chapter
- All the official ICD-10-CM codes, indexes, notes, footnotes, and symbols
- Icons and definitions to differentiate between the two types of Excludes notes
- Check 4th, 5th, 6th, and 7th character symbols that identify codes that require the addition of a 4th, 5th, 6th, or 7th character for code specificity and validity
- Color coding and symbol legend at the bottom of each page

Please review "How to Use *ICD-10-CM Professional for Physicians*" in this section to learn about the features that will help you assign and report correct codes, ensuring appropriate reimbursement.

# How to Use ICD-10-CM Professional for Physicians 2018

This International Classification of Diseases, 10th Revision, Clinical Modification (ICD-10-CM) is being published by the United States Government in recognition of its responsibility to promulgate this classification throughout the United States for morbidity coding. This code book represents an adaptation of ICD-10 that was created specifically for use in the United States. Revisions to ICD-10-CM will be made based on the established update process for ICD-10-CM (the ICD-10-CM Coordination and Maintenance Committee) and the World Health Organization's ICD-10 (the Update and Revision Committee).

## Use of Official Sources

The *ICD-10-CM Professional for Physicians* contains the official U.S. Department of Health and Human Services, Tenth Revision, Clinical Modification, ICD-10-CM codes, effective for the current year.

Much of the color coding and many of the symbols that identify coding and reimbursement issues are derived from official federal government sources, including the Integrated Outpatient Code Editor (IOCE), version 18.2.

For the most current IOCE documents please refer to the following: https://www.cms.gov/Medicare/Coding/OutpatientCodeEdit/OCEQtrReleaseSpecs.html.

## Steps to Correct Coding

1. Before beginning to use this code book, review section I.A., "Conventions for the ICD-10-CM," and section I.B., "General Coding Guidelines," of the ICD-10-CM Official Guidelines for Coding and Reporting.

2. Look up the main term in the alphabetic index and scan the subterm entries as appropriate. Review continued lines and additional subterms that may appear in the next column or on the next page.

3. Note all parenthetical terms (nonessential modifiers) that help in code selection but do not affect code assignment. Shaded vertical guidelines in the index are provided to help determine the indentation level for each subterm in relation to the main terms.

4. Pay close attention to the following instructions in the index:

   – "See," "see also," and "see category" cross-references

   – "With"/"without" notes

   – "Omit code" notes

   – "Due to" subterms

   – Other instructions found in note boxes, such as "code by site"

   – *Following* references and Check Additional Character symbol in the indexes. The *following* references (designed and used exclusively by Optum360) help coders locate those alphanumeric codes that are out of sequence in the tabular section.

5. Do not code from the alphabetic index without verifying the accuracy of the code in the tabular list. Locate the code in the alphanumerically arranged tabular list.

6. To determine the appropriateness of the code selection and proper coding, read all instructional material:

   – "Includes" and both types of "Excludes" notes

   – "Use additional code" and "code first underlying disease" instructions

   – "Code also"

   – 4th, 5th, and 6th character requirements and 7th character extension requirements

   – Age and sex symbols

7. Consult the official ICD-10-CM guidelines, which govern the use of specific codes. These guidelines provide both general and chapter-specific coding guidance.

8. Confirm and assign the correct code.

## Organization

This book is organized in the following manner:

### Introduction

The introductory material in this book includes the ICD-10-CM Official Preface, the history of ICD-10-CM as well as an overview of the classification system.

### Official ICD-10-CM Conventions and Guidelines

This section provides an explanation of the conventions and guidelines regulating the appropriate assignment and reporting of ICD-10-CM codes. This coding guidance is presented by the National Center for Health Statistics (NCHS), a governmental agency of the Centers for Disease Control and Prevention (CDC), within the United States Department of Health and Human Services (DHHS). **Note: The 2018 *ICD-10-CM Official Guidelines for Coding and Reporting* were not available at the time this book went to print. Updated guidelines will be posted on our website at https://www.optum360coding.com/ProductUpdates/ as soon as they are available.**

### Alphabetic Index to Diseases

The Alphabetic Index to Diseases is arranged in alphabetic order by disease — by specific illness, injury, eponym, abbreviation, or other descriptive diagnostic term. The Index also lists diagnostic terms for other reasons for encounters with health care professionals.

### Neoplasm Table

The Neoplasm Table provides the proper code based upon histology of the neoplasm and site.

### Table of Drugs and Chemicals

The Table of Drugs and Chemicals lists the drug and the specific codes that identify the drug and the intent. No additional external cause of injury and poisoning code is assigned in ICD-10-CM.

### Index to External Causes

The Alphabetic Index to External Causes of Injuries is arranged in alphabetic order by main term indicating the event.

### Tabular List of Diseases

ICD-10-CM codes and descriptors are arranged numerically within the tabular list of diseases within 21 separate chapters according to body system or nature of injury and disease. Classifications that were previously considered supplemental to ICD-9-CM (e.g., V codes and E codes) are incorporated into the tabular listing of ICD-10-CM as individual chapters. Chapters 20, "External Causes of Morbidity," and 21, "Factors Influencing Health Status and Contact with Health Services," include chapter-specific guidelines.

### Illustrations

This section includes illustrations of normal anatomy with ICD-10-CM specific terminology.

# Overview of ICD-10-CM Official Conventions

This is an overview of the ICD-10-CM official conventions, which are general rules for using the classification system, independent of the guidelines. The official conventions and instructions of the classification, which take precedence over the guidelines, are incorporated within the alphabetic index and tabular list as instructional notes and are applicable regardless of the health care setting. For the full version of the official conventions, see the ICD-10-CM Official Guidelines for Coding and Reporting, section I.A., which is included in this book.

## Format

ICD-10-CM is divided into two main parts: the index, an alphabetical list of terms and their corresponding code, and the tabular list, a sequential, alphanumeric list of codes divided into chapters based on body system or condition. The index contains the Index to Diseases and Injuries (main index) and the Index to External Causes of Injury. Also included in the main index is the Neoplasm Table and a Table of Drugs and Chemicals.

The tabular list contains categories, subcategories, and valid codes. ICD-10-CM is an alphanumeric classification system. The 1st character of a three-character category is a letter. The 2nd and 3rd characters may be numbers or alpha characters. A three-character category without further subclassification is equivalent to a valid three-character code. Subcategories are either four or five characters. Subcategory characters include either letters or numbers. Codes may be three, four, five, six, or seven characters in length, in which each level of subdivision after a category is a subcategory. The final level of subdivision is a valid code. The final character in a code may be either a letter or a number.

The ICD-10-CM uses the letter "X" as a placeholder. A placeholder "X" is used as a 5th character placeholder at certain six-character codes to allow for future expansion, without disturbing the 6th character structure. For instance, an initial encounter for accidental poisoning by penicillin is coded to T36.0X1A. The "X" in the 5th character position is a placeholder, or filler character.

Similarly, certain categories have applicable 7th character extensions. In these cases, the 7th character extension is required for all codes within the category, or as otherwise instructed in the tabular list notations. 7th character extensions must always be the last character in the data field. If a code is not a full six characters in length, a dummy placeholder "X" must be used to fill in the empty characters when a 7th character extension is required.

## Punctuation

[ ]   In the tabular list, brackets are used to enclose synonyms, alternative wording, or explanatory phrases. In the index, brackets are used to identify manifestation codes.

( )   Parentheses are used in both the index and tabular list to enclose nonessential modifiers; supplementary words that may be present or absent in the statement of a disease or procedure without affecting the code number to which it is assigned.

:   Colons are used in the tabular list after an incomplete term that needs one or more of the modifiers following the colon to make it assignable to a given category.

## Abbreviations

### NEC

The abbreviation NEC, "Not elsewhere classifiable" represents "other specified" in the ICD-10-CM. An index entry that states NEC directs the coder to an "other specified" code in the tabular list. Codes titled "Other" or "Other specified" in the tabular list (usually a code with a 4th or 6th character 8 and 5th character 9) are for use when the information in the medical record provides detail for which a specific code does not exist.

### NOS

The abbreviation NOS, "Not otherwise specified," in the tabular list may be interpreted as "unspecified." Codes in the tabular list with "Unspecified" in the title (usually a code with a 4th or 6th character 9 and 5th character 0) are for use when the information in the medical record is insufficient to assign a more specific code.

## Typeface

### Boldface

Boldface type is used for main term entries in the alphabetic index, and all codes and descriptions in the tabular list.

## General Notes

The following conventions and notes appear only in the tabular list of diseases:

### Includes Notes

The word INCLUDES appears immediately under certain categories to further define, clarify, or give examples of the content of a code category.

### Inclusion Terms

Lists of inclusion terms are included under certain codes. These terms indicate some of the conditions for which that code number may be used. Inclusion terms may be synonyms with the code title, or, in the case of "other specified" codes, the terms may also provide a list of various conditions included within a classification code. The inclusion terms are not exhaustive. The index may provide additional terms that may also be assigned to a given code.

### Excludes Notes

ICD-10-CM has two types of excludes notes. Each note has a different definition for use. However, they are similar in that they both indicate that codes excluded from each other are independent of each other.

### Excludes 1

An EXCLUDES 1 note is a "pure" excludes. It means "NOT CODED HERE!" An Excludes 1 note indicates mutually exclusive codes: two conditions that cannot be reported together. For example, a congenital form of a disease may not be reported with the acquired form of the same condition. The code excluded should never be reported with the applicable codes listed above the excludes notation.

An exception to the Excludes 1 definition is when the two conditions are unrelated to each other. If it is not clear whether the two conditions involving an Excludes 1 note are related or not, query the provider. For example, code F45.8 Other somatoform disorders, has an Excludes 1 note for "sleep related teeth grinding (G47.63)" because "teeth grinding" is an inclusion term under F45.8. Only one of these two codes should be assigned for teeth grinding. However psychogenic dysmenorrhea is also an inclusion term under F45.8, and a patient could have both this condition and sleep-related teeth grinding. In this case, the two conditions are clearly unrelated to each other, so it would be appropriate to report F45.8 and G47.63 together.

## Excludes 2

An EXCLUDES 2 note means "NOT INCLUDED HERE." An Excludes 2 note indicates that although the excluded condition is not part of the condition it is excluded from, a patient may have both conditions at the same time. Therefore, when an Excludes 2 note appears under a code, it may be acceptable to use both the code and the excluded code together if supported by the medical documentation.

## Note

NOTE The term "NOTE" appears as an icon and precedes the instructional information. These notes function as alerts to highlight coding instructions within the text.

## Default Codes

In the index, the default code is the code listed next to the main term. The default code represents the condition most commonly associated with the main term. This code may be assigned when documentation does not facilitate reporting a more specific code. Alternatively, it may provide an unspecified code for the condition.

## Syndromes

Follow the alphabetic index guidance when coding syndromes. In the absence of index guidance, assign codes for the documented manifestations of the syndrome.

## And

When the term "and" is used in a narrative statement or code title it may be interpreted as "and/or."

## With

The word "with" should be interpreted to mean "associated with" or "due to" when it appears in a code title, the Alphabetic Index, or an instructional note in the Tabular List. The classification presumes a causal relationship between the two conditions linked by these terms in the Alphabetic Index or Tabular List. These conditions should be coded as related even in the absence of provider documentation explicitly linking them, unless the documentation clearly states the conditions are unrelated. For conditions not specifically linked by these relational terms in the classification, provider documentation must link the conditions in order to code them as related. The word "with" in the Alphabetic Index is sequenced immediately following the main term, not in alphabetical order.

## See and See Also

When the instruction "See" follows a main term in the alphabetic index, it indicates that another term must be referenced in order to locate the correct code. The instructional note "See also" simply provides alternative terms that may be useful in determining the correct code but is not necessary to follow if the main term supplies the appropriate code.

## Instructional Notes Used in the Tabular List

In the tabular section, the following instructional notes appear in red type for emphasis:

## Code First/Use additional code:

These instructional notes provide sequencing instruction. They may appear independently of each other or to designate certain etiology/manifestation paired codes. These instructions signal the coder that an additional code should be reported to provide a more complete picture of that diagnosis.

In etiology/manifestation coding, ICD-10-CM requires the underlying condition to be sequenced first, followed by the manifestation. In these situations, codes with "In diseases classified elsewhere" in the code description are never permitted as a first-listed or principal diagnosis code and must be sequenced following the underlying condition code.

## Code Also:

A "code also" note alerts the coder that more than one code may be required to fully describe the condition. Code sequencing is discretionary. Factors that may determine sequencing include severity and reason for the encounter.

## Code Assignment and Clinical Criteria

Diagnosis code assignment must be based on the provider's diagnostic statement that the condition exists and is not based on clinical criteria the provider used to establish the diagnosis. Conflicting documentation must be queried.

# Additional Annotations

## Code-Level Notations

The tabular section of ICD-10-CM has various colors, symbols, and other tabular annotations that may help in code selection, provide clinical or coding information, or alert the coder to reimbursement issues affected by the diagnosis code assignment. Some codes may have more than one annotation. For quick reference to the meanings of the colors and symbols, look at the color/symbol legend at the bottom of each page in the tabular list.

## Italics

Italicized type is used for all exclusion notes and to identify manifestation codes, those codes that should not be reported as first-listed (principal) diagnoses.

## Color Coding/Symbols

### New Code

This ● icon identifies the codes that are new to the classification system for the current year. The new code icon is to the left of the code.

### Revised Code Title

This ▲ icon to the left of a code alerts the user to a change in that code's title. This change may be as simple as adding or removing punctuation, which may or may not change the intent of the code, to adding or removing specific terms from a code description that completely alter the circumstances in which the code would be used.

### Revised Text

The revised text ►◄ "bow ties" alert the user to changes in parenthetical notes for the current year. Revised text may include the following:

- A change in a current parenthetical description

- A change in the code(s) associated with a current parenthetical note

- A change in how a current parenthetical note is classified (e.g., an Excludes 1 note that changes to an Excludes 2 note)

- Addition of a new parenthetical note(s) to a code

### Deleted Text

Strikethrough on code description(s) and/or code note(s) indicates a deletion from the classification for the current year. For example:

**✓4ᵗʰ N25  Disorders resulting from impaired renal tubular function**
       **EXCLUDES 1**  ~~metabolic disorders classifiable to E70-E88~~

The strikethrough over the Excludes 1 note indicates that this note was deleted from the classification and is no longer applicable to codes in category N25.

      **✓7ᵗʰ  S63.131  ~~Subluxation of proximal interphalangeal joint of right thumb~~**

The strikethrough over the code and the code description indicates that all codes in subcategory S63.131 (S63.131A, S63.131D, and S63.131S) have been deleted from the classification.

### Additional Characters Required

**✓4ᵗʰ** This symbol indicates that the code requires a 4th character.

**✓5ᵗʰ** This symbol indicates that the code requires a 5th character.

**✓6ᵗʰ** This symbol indicates that the code requires a 6th character.

**✓7ᵗʰ** This symbol indicates that the code requires a 7th character.

**✓x7ᵗʰ** This symbol indicates that the code requires a 7th character following the placeholder "X." Codes with fewer than six characters

that require a 7th character must contain placeholder "X" to fill in the empty character(s).

### Key Word

Green font is used throughout the Tabular List of Diseases to differentiate the key words that appear in similar code descriptions in a given category or subcategory.

For example, refer to the list of codes below from category C7A:

C7A.020  Malignant carcinoid tumor of the **appendix**

C7A.021  Malignant carcinoid tumor of the **cecum**

C7A.022  Malignant carcinoid tumor of the **ascending colon**

C7A.023  Malignant carcinoid tumor of the **transverse colon**

C7A.024  Malignant carcinoid tumor of the **descending colon**

C7A.025  Malignant carcinoid tumor of the **sigmoid colon**

C7A.026  Malignant carcinoid tumor of the **rectum**

C7A.029  Malignant carcinoid tumor of the large intestine, unspecified portion

The portion of the code description that appears in **green font** in the tabular list assists the coder in quickly identifying the key terms and in identifying the correct code. This convention is especially useful when the codes describe laterality, such as the following codes from subcategory H40.22:

H40.221  Chronic angle-closure glaucoma, **right** eye

H40.222  Chronic angle-closure glaucoma, **left** eye

H40.223  Chronic angle-closure glaucoma, **bilateral**

H40.229  Chronic angle-closure glaucoma, unspecified eye

The key word convention is used only in those categories in which there are multiple codes with very similar descriptions with only a few words that differentiate them.

### Medicare Code Edits

Medicare Administrative Contractors and many payers use Medicare code edits to check the coding accuracy on claims. The coding edit information in this manual reflects those edits used for outpatient institutional providers, which also include hospitals that are subject to the outpatient prospective payment system (OPPS). These edits have been updated to reflect changes in the Integrated Outpatient Code Editor (IOCE), version 18.2.

#### *Manifestation Code*

These codes appear in italic type, with a **blue color bar** over the title. A manifestation code cannot be reported as a first-listed or principal diagnosis. By definition, a manifestation code represents a demonstration of some aspect of an underlying disease, which is separately classifiable. In the alphabetic index, these codes are listed as the secondary code in brackets. The underlying disease code is listed first.

#### *Age and Sex Edit*

The age and sex edits below are used to detect inconsistencies between the patient's age and/or sex and the patient's diagnosis. The following edit symbols appear in the tabular list to the right of the code description.

**Newborn Age: 0**                                                                 Ⓝ

    These diagnoses are intended for newborns and neonates and the patient's age must be 0 years.

**Additional Annotations**

### Pediatric Age: 0-17

☐P

These diagnoses are intended for children and the patient's age must be between 0 and 17 years.

### Maternity Age: 12-55

☐M

These diagnoses are intended for childbearing patients between the age of 12 and 55 years.

### Adult Age: 15-124

☐A

These diagnoses are intended for patients between the age of 15 and 124 years.

### Male diagnosis only

♂

### Female diagnosis only

♀

## Medicare Advantage Risk Adjustment Edits

Medicare Advantage plans provided as part of the Medicare Part C program use a risk-adjustment model to plan for future healthcare costs of Medicare Part C participants. The risk-adjustment model measures disease burden by assigning certain ICD-10-CM diagnosis codes to hierarchical condition categories (HCC). The HCC information in this manual has been updated to reflect the CMS-HCC model category for v22 of the CMS-HCC risk-adjustment software.

### HCC

HCC

This symbol indicates that the condition is considered a CMS-HCC diagnosis. All HCC conditions that are appropriately documented are used in the risk-adjustment model for Medicare Advantage to provide a means of comparing quality of care across Medicare Part C participants as well as predict future healthcare costs.

The HCC icon appears to the right of the code description.

## Other Code-Level Notations

### Unspecified Code

▽

Use these codes when neither the diagnostic statement nor the documentation provides enough information to assign a more specific diagnosis code. These codes may be stated as "Unspecified" or "Not otherwise specified (NOS)."

**Note:** Do not assign these codes when a more specific diagnosis has been determined.

### PDx Symbol

PDx

This symbol identifies a Z code that generally is for use as a first-listed (or principal) diagnosis only but may be used as an additional diagnosis if the patient has more than one encounter on the same day or there is more than one reason for the encounter.

The instructions for Z code use contained in the ICD-10-CM official coding guidelines identify those Z codes that can be used only as a PDx. All other Z codes may either be SDx or PDx, depending upon circumstances of the encounter, by meeting the definition of first-listed or principal diagnosis, and by following any specific Z code guidelines in section I.C.21 a-c. The responsibility of those assigning the Z codes as PDx is to make sure the circumstances of the encounter meet the definition of first-listed or principal diagnosis, follow all coding instructions, and follow the Z code specific guidelines. Optum360 does not include any SDx edit since there is no official source for it and the Z code use is determined by circumstances of the encounter.

**Note:** Please note that the symbols indicating the Z code "principal or first-listed only" designation and the Z codes that may be principal or first-listed diagnoses included in the official coding guidelines [Section I.C.21.c.16] are consistent with reporting guidelines for health care encounters *excluding acute care inpatient admissions*. These Z code edits are often in conflict with the inpatient prospective payment system (IPPS) edits. For example, code Z34.90 Encounter for supervision of normal pregnancy, unspecified, unspecified trimester, may be an appropriate primary reason for an outpatient encounter. However, supervision for a normal pregnancy is not an acceptable principal diagnosis or reason for an inpatient admission and will have an unacceptable principal diagnosis edit under the inpatient prospective payment system (IPPS).

### AHA:

This symbol precedes official citations from AHA's *Coding Clinic for ICD-10-CM/PCS*. Similar to the parenthetical notes, AHA references are placed in a hierarchical pattern at the chapter, code block, category, subcategory, or valid code level. This means that the information found in the reference applies to one or more codes depending on where the citation is placed.

The citations appear in purple type and are listed with the most current citation first. *Coding Clinic* citations included in this edition have been updated through second quarter 2017.

### DEF:

This symbol precedes a definition of a condition or disease.

The definition appears in purple type directly under the code.

### TIP:

This symbol precedes coding advice that is not readily available within the ICD-10-CM classification. It may relate official coding guidelines, indexing nuances, or advice from *AHA's Coding Clinic for ICD-10-CM/PCS*.

The tip appears in purple type directly under the code.

## Footnotes

All footnotes are identified by a numerical superscript that appears to the upper left of the code. For example:

[1] ✓x7th **M48.50 Collapsed vertebra, not elsewhere classified, site unspecified** HCC

The footnote 1 indicates "HCC with 7th character indicating initial encounter." This means that a collapsed vertebra would be considered an HCC only when the 7th character represents an initial encounter, such as 7th character A, B, or C, depending on the category.

The following list identifies the meaning of each footnote number in the Tabular List of Diseases:

1    These codes are considered an HCC when reported with a 7th character indicating an initial encounter (7th character A, B, or C).

2    These codes are considered an HCC when reported with a 7th character indicating an initial encounter (7th character A or B) OR sequela.

3    These codes are considered an HCC when reported with a 7th character indicating sequela.

# Chapter-Level Notations

## Chapter-Specific Guidelines with Coding Examples

Each chapter begins with the Official Guidelines for Coding and Reporting specific to that chapter, where provided. Coding examples, specific to outpatient care settings, have been provided to illustrate the coding and/or sequencing guidance in these guidelines.

## Muscle and Tendon Table

ICD-10-CM categorizes certain muscles and tendons in the upper and lower extremities by their action (e.g., extension or flexion) as well as their anatomical location. The Muscle/Tendon table is provided at the beginning of chapter 13 and chapter 19 to help users when code selection depends on the action of the muscle and/or tendon.

**Note:** This table is not all-inclusive, and proper code assignment should be based on the provider's documentation.

## Index Notations

▽ Subterms under main terms may continue to next column or page. This warning statement is a reminder to always check for additional subterms and information that may continue onto the next page or column before making a final selection.

### *Following* References

The index includes *following* references to assist in locating "out-of-sequence" codes in the tabular list. "Out-of-sequence" codes contain an alphabetic character (letter) in the 3rd or 4th character position. These codes are placed according to the classification rules — the placement of the codes according to condition — not according to alphabetic or numeric sequencing rules.

*Examples:*

**Carcinoma (malignant)** (*see also,* Neoplasm, by site, malignant)
    neuroendocrine (*see also* Tumor, neuroendocrine)

    high grade, any site C7A.1 (*following* C75)
    poorly differentiated, any site C7A.1 (*following* C75)

In the tabular rubric, C7A is included after rubric C75 and before C76.

**Gout, chronic** (*see also* Gout, gouty) M1A.9
    drug-induced M1A.20 (*following* M08)
        ankle M1A.27-(*following* M08)
        elbow M1A.22-(*following* M08)

In the tabular rubric, M1A is included after rubric M08 and before M10.